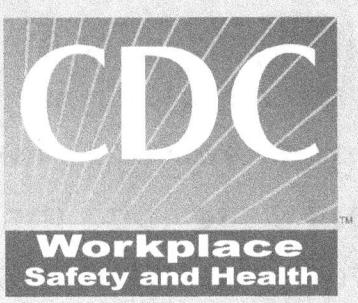

I0426408

Evaluation of Resident Aggression Toward Staff in a Center for the Developmentally Disabled – Michigan

Christine West, RN, MSN/MPH
Ellen Galloway, MA

Health Hazard Evaluation Report
HETA 2008-0046-3123
March 2011

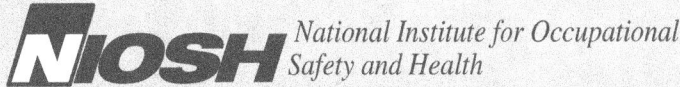

DEPARTMENT OF HEALTH AND HUMAN SERVICES
Centers for Disease Control and Prevention

NIOSH *National Institute for Occupational Safety and Health*

The employer shall post a copy of this report for a period of 30 calendar days at or near the workplace(s) of affected employees. The employer shall take steps to insure that the posted determinations are not altered, defaced, or covered by other material during such period. [37 FR 23640, November 7, 1972, as amended at 45 FR 2653, January 14, 1980].

CONTENTS

ABBREVIATIONS

BLS	Bureau of Labor Statistics
HHE	Health hazard evaluation
ICF/MR	Intermediate Care Facility for the Mentally Retarded
IPP	Individual Program Plan
NAICS	North American Industry Classification System
NIOSH	National Institute for Occupational Safety and Health
OSHA	Occupational Safety and Health Administration
PPD	Personal protective device

Highlights of the NIOSH Health Hazard Evaluation

The National Institute for Occupational Safety and Health (NIOSH) received a request for a health hazard evaluation from the management of an intermediate care facility for the mentally retarded (ICF/MR) in Michigan. The request was made because staff were being injured in assaults by residents. This center has closed since our evaluation.

What NIOSH Did

- We toured the center on July 8-9, 2008, and observed work areas. We talked with direct care staff about their health, their jobs, and resident aggression.

- We calculated injury rates based on Occupational Safety and Health Administration Logs for 2004-2008. These rates were then compared with national rates.

- We reviewed the Michigan Interpretive Guidelines for Intermediate Care Facilities for Persons with Mental Retardation. We also looked at the center's plan for controlling exposures to bloodborne pathogens.

What NIOSH Found

- Center staff were at risk of injury from assault by residents.

- Many staff thought that management lacked concern about their safety.

- Staff reported that most injuries occurred while physically restraining residents.

- The injury and illness incidence rate associated with assault was higher than national rates for healthcare and social assistance centers.

- The facility lacked policies and procedures to support a safe and nonviolent workplace.

- The plan for controlling exposures to bloodborne pathogens did not take into account the risk of infectious diseases associated with assaults by residents.

What Managers Can Do

- Form a safety committee that will develop a safety program to address safety issues at the facility. The program should also create a safety climate that is responsive to resident and staff needs.

- Create a human rights committee to address issues of resident aggression. This is required by the Michigan Interpretive Guidelines for Intermediate Care Facilities for Persons with Mental Retardation.

- Hire additional staff to provide a higher staff-to-resident ratio to help prevent incidents of aggression.

- Teach staff how to deal with resident aggression effectively.

Highlights of the NIOSH Health Hazard Evaluation (continued)

What Employees Can Do

- Wear clothing such as jeans and long sleeves to help protect from bites and other injuries.

- Remove objects in the environment that could be used as weapons.

- Report all injuries to a supervisor and seek care from a healthcare provider.

- Talk about aggression during program planning meetings for residents.

- Become active in safety and human rights committees.

- Take part in training on how to deal with resident aggression and strategies for self-care.

Summary

Direct care and nursing staff at this ICF/MR were at risk of injury from assault by residents. Although the center is now closed, we recommend that management at similar facilities develop a workplace violence program that has full participation of employees and managers and is evaluated periodically.

In November 2007, NIOSH received an HHE request from management of an ICF/MR, a center for the developmentally disabled, in Michigan. The request was submitted because of a high number of injuries among staff from resident aggression.

On July 8–9, 2008, we visited the center, where we held an opening conference and met with management. We also held employee interviews, reviewed records and procedures, and toured each of the buildings at the center.

Residents' apartments appeared crowded with furniture. In some instances, residents would not be in clear sight of the staff when few staff were working. Staff reported that the personal alarms for alerting coworkers to respond to an incident site did not work in all locations. We observed no other alarm systems or communication devices on site.

We interviewed 24 direct care workers and nursing staff who reported being injured by a resident, and most reported being injured while physically restraining patients. These employees reported that an inadequate number of staff responded to events. They also reported that managers lacked concern about their safety and that they did not feel managers would heed their suggestions about how to handle resident aggression. In addition, they reported that they were not fully included in the residents' IPP process. Half of the staff expressed a need for more comprehensive training on handling resident aggression.

The number of injuries and illnesses reported on the OSHA Form 300 Log of Work-Related Injuries and Illnesses increased from 2004 to 2006. Nonfatal injury and illness incidence rates were approximately three times higher than national rates in nursing and residential care facilities in 2004 and 2005. Most injuries were from assault, and the number of assault injuries increased over time. The incidence rates of assaults were higher than national rates for the nursing and social assistance sector from 2004 to 2008, with the highest rate occurring in 2006. The most common injuries related to resident assaults were strains/sprains, bruises, and bites. Of the workers' compensation claims, 13 (of 35) were filed by staff who assisted in physically restraining aggressive residents.

The facility provided no written policies or procedures on workplace violence. Managers reported that during new employee

SUMMARY
(CONTINUED)

orientation and annually thereafter, direct care staff completed crisis intervention training, which focuses on handling agitated behaviors and applying physical restraint. Our review of the ICF/MR regulations showed that in several instances, the center did not follow the regulations on staffing ratios, convening a human rights committee, proper use of medication to manage resident behavior, and staff training. The plan for controlling exposure to bloodborne pathogens did not take into account the risk of infectious diseases from resident assaults.

Although the center has closed since our evaluation, we feel that the results of this evaluation may benefit any ICF/MR or other similar facility. We encourage such facilities to develop a safety and health program that includes management and employee participation, hazard identification, safety and health training, and hazard prevention, control, and reporting. Employers should evaluate this program periodically. Our recommendations are based on the general violence-prevention strategies outlined in the document OSHA Guidelines for Preventing Workplace Violence for Health Care & Social Service Workers [OSHA 2004].

Keywords: NAICS 622210 (Psychiatric and Substance Abuse Hospitals), ICF/MR, workplace violence, injury

INTRODUCTION

On November 27, 2007, NIOSH received an HHE request from the management of a Michigan ICF/MR, a center for the developmentally disabled. NIOSH was asked to identify risk factors for resident aggressive and violent behavior toward direct care staff and to provide recommendations to decrease assaults. We visited the center on July 8–9, 2008, and met with managers, employees, and representatives from two unions; toured the facility; and interviewed staff.

Background

The center was a Michigan-operated ICF/MR for persons with developmental disabilities and/or mental illness. After the evaluation, we were notified that the facility was closing and all residents were being transferred to family members' homes, group homes, or other facilities. The center's residents lived in a series of buildings split into four sex-segregated apartments. The apartments contained common areas for residents to eat, watch television, play games, and engage in other activities. Residents gathered for activities or participated in treatment in the common areas and in other buildings at the center. One building housed people with mental and physical disabilities who required extensive care and assistance with all activities of daily living. Many used wheelchairs and had substantial functional limitations. Two buildings housed able-bodied individuals with mental retardation and/or mental illness. A fourth building housed people who had been admitted to the center from the court system because they had pled not guilty by reason of insanity to a crime. These last three buildings included residents with mild mental retardation and/or mental illness who were able-bodied and moved freely around their apartments and the center's grounds. Admission to the center was considered only when no local resources or less restrictive residential options were available. Some residents were placed at the center because of their aggressive behavior.

At the time of our evaluation, the center employed 251 resident care aides and nursing, medical, and therapy staff; and 158 administrative, housekeeping, and maintenance staff. The largest groups of employees at the center were resident care aides, licensed practical nurses, and registered nurses. The U.S. Department of Labor defines direct care workers as nursing aides, orderlies, and attendants in any setting (institutional or residential). Similarly, in this evaluation, we refer to resident care aides as direct care workers. Because of the nature of their work, nurses and direct care workers had the most contact with residents; they provided for the residents' physical, medical, and habilitation needs as specified in their IPPs. Nurses and direct care employees worked one of three 8-hour shifts to provide 24-hour staffing of the center. Overtime was needed to cover understaffed shifts. Those who wished to volunteer for overtime used a sign-up sheet in the break room, but supervisors assigned mandatory overtime to staff for uncovered shifts. Typically, staff worked one 8-hour overtime shift per week.

ASSESSMENT

We visited the center July 8-9, 2008. We toured the buildings; observed the settings and staff interactions with residents in buildings 405, 608, 609, and 610; and interviewed nurses and direct care workers. Before our visit, we obtained copies of the OSHA Form 300 Log of Work-Related Injuries and Illnesses from the period 2004–2008 and a list of employees who received assault-related workers' compensation during the period of June 2006 to May 2008.

Health Interviews

From a staffing list of direct care workers, licensed practical nurses, and registered nurses from all three shifts, we serially selected employees for interviews. In addition, employees who were interested in an interview were invited to participate. We collected the following information: name, age, job duration, usual shift, medical history, extent of overtime, injuries from resident assault, circumstances that led to acts of aggression and possible injury, management perceptions of resident aggression, existing policies, and training programs designed to reduce resident aggression.

OSHA Logs and Workers' Compensation Claims

From the OSHA Log data, we calculated nonfatal injury and illness incidence rates and compared them with national incidence rates for nursing and residential care facilities for 2004–2008 (NAICS code: 623000). On the basis of incident reports, management identified injuries on the OSHA Logs that were caused by assault. We also calculated the incidence rate of injuries due to assault and compared these to rates for the healthcare and social assistance sector for 2004–2008 (NAICS code: 62). National assault incidence rates were not available for nursing and residential care facilities. For these calculations and comparisons, we used a formula available on the BLS website, at http://data.bls.gov/IIRC/calculate.do. Incidence rates represent the number of injuries and/or illnesses per 100 full-time workers and were calculated as follows:

$$N/EH \times 200,000$$

where

N = number of injuries and illnesses/injuries due to assault,

EH = total number of hours worked by all center employees during the calendar year, and

200,000 = base for 100 full-time-equivalent workers (working 40 hours per week, 50 weeks per year).

Policy and Training Document Review

We reviewed the Michigan Interpretive Guidelines for Intermediate Care Facilities for Persons with Mental Retardation and the center's control plan for bloodborne pathogen exposure. We also reviewed employee training requirements for intervening in and managing inappropriate resident behavior.

RESULTS

Observations

In buildings 405, 609, and 610, male and female residents lived in separate apartments with communal bedrooms, living room, kitchen, and small activity room. Residents engaged in scheduled activities in nonresidential building 608, which had a large common area. The apartments were adequately lit and contained few loose objects that could be used as weapons. We observed no sharp objects or items that contained glass other than a few wall clocks. The apartments contained plastic or heavy wooden furniture, and some rooms appeared crowded. We observed several rooms and hallways where residents would not be in clear sight of the staff when few staff were working. Staff carried a PPD, a personal alarm that if activated would signal other staff to respond to that location during an incident. Staff reported that the PPDs did not work in all locations inside and outside the buildings and that, at times, not enough people responded to the incident for assistance. We observed no other alarm system or communication devices on site.

Staff Interviews

We interviewed 20 direct care workers, two licensed practical nurses, one registered nurse, and one direct care supervisor. Table 1 summarizes the demographics and responses of the interviewees.

All staff members interviewed reported that they had been injured by residents and that work-related injuries from resident aggression had been increasing; 20 (83%) reported being injured while engaged in physical restraint of a resident. Half reported needing to see a healthcare provider for their injuries, and slightly fewer than half requested time off work for their injuries. Several staff showed us lacerations and bruises from resident aggression. When asked to identify factors that contributed to injury from patient aggression, 10 staff (42%) said that the number of staff responding to an incident was typically insufficient, and 20 staff (83%) reported that managers lacked concern about their safety and would not consider their suggestions about how to handle resident aggression. Of the staff interviewed, 13 (54%) reported that they were not fully included in the residents' IPP process, including providing input to the medical provider about behavior that might warrant changes in the residents' medication. They reported that medication reductions seemed to result in resident aggression. Half of the staff expressed a need for more comprehensive training on handling resident aggression.

Table 1. Demographics and responses of the center's direct care staff who were interviewed (N = 24)

Characteristic	Variable	No.	%
Sex	Women	19	79
Job title	Resident Care Aide	21	88
	Licensed Practical Nurse	2	8
	Registered Nurse	1	4
Work shift	Morning	11	46
	Afternoon	10	42
	Midnight	3	13
Work duration	< 5 years	5	21
	5–10 years	13	54
	>10 years	6	25
Overtime	Yes	20	83
	Mandatory	12	50
	Voluntary	8	33
	No	4	17
Injured in assault by resident	Yes	24	100
	Consulted healthcare provider	12	50
	Time off work	11	46
	No	0	0
Injured during physical restraint of resident	Yes	20	83
	Inadequate staff responding to incident	10	42
	Lack of concern about staff safety	20	83
	Lack of input into resident IPP	13	54
	Inadequate training on handling resident aggression	12	50

OSHA Logs and Workers' Compensation Claims

Table 2 presents the number of injuries and illnesses recorded in the OSHA Log and compares incidence rates of nonfatal injuries and illnesses at the center with national incidence rates for nursing and residential care facilities from 2004 to 2008. OSHA Log data were available for the first 6 months of 2008. The number of injuries and illnesses increased from 2004 to 2007. Incidence rates for injuries and illnesses increased from 2004 to 2006, with a slight decrease in 2007. Nonfatal injury and illness incidence rates were approximately three times higher than national rates in nursing and residential care facilities in 2004 and 2005. In 2006 and 2007, rates at the center were approximately four to five times higher than national rates.

Table 2. Number of nonfatal injury and illness cases and incidence rates from OSHA logs for 2004–2008 at the center, compared with national rates

Variable	2004	2005	2006	2007	2008*
No. of injury and illness cases at the center	131	143	204	162	54
Injury and illness incidence rates† at the center	26	31	41.3	37.5	13
National incidence rates† for nursing and residential care facilities	9.7	9.1	8.9	8.8	8.4

*Data available for January–June 2008.
†Per 100 full-time employees.

Table 3 presents the number of injuries due to assault, assault incidence rates at the center, and national incidence rates in the healthcare and social assistance sector. Most injuries represented in Table 2 were caused by assault; injuries due to assault increased over time except for a slight decrease in 2007. Assault incidence rates were higher than national assault rates for the nursing and social assistance sector during the period 2004–2008, with the highest rate occurring in 2006. Most assault injuries resulted in no missed work days from 2004 through 2008. For those injuries due to assault that did result in days lost, a total of 3,382 lost work days were recorded during the 2004–2008 period.

Table 3. Number of injuries from assault cases and incidence rates from OSHA logs for 2004–2008 at the center, compared with national rates

Variable	2004	2005	2006	2007	2008*
No. of cases due to assault at the center	85	92	140	121	40
Assault incidence rates† at the center	17	20	32.4	29	9.3
National incidence rates† of assaults in health care and social assistance	0.11	0.84	0.83	0.83	0.82

*Data available for January–June 2008.
†Per 100 full-time employees.

RESULTS
(CONTINUED)

Table 4 presents the types of injuries resulting from assault for 2004–2008. Overall, the most common injuries related to resident assaults over the 4-year period were strains/sprains, bruises, bites, head trauma, broken bones, and lacerations. Some recorded incidents involved multiple injuries. Resident care aide was the most common job type reported with injuries due to assault.

Table 4. Types (numbers) of injuries related to resident assaults at the center, from OSHA logs, 2004–2008

Variable	2004	2005	2006	2007	2008*
Strains/sprains	52	30	45	38	20
Contusions	17	31	36	26	6
Bites	9	10	34	36	9
Head trauma/injury	5	4	4	7	2
Fractures	3	2	1	4	1
Lacerations/scratches/abrasions	2	5	8	6	2
Facial injuries	2	5	8	2	4
Other	3	6	5	5	1

*Data available for January–June 2008.

From June 2006 to May 2008, 35 workers' compensation claims were paid for injuries involving a resident assault encounter. Of these, 22 injuries occurred as a result of resident aggression and 13 occurred to staff who assisted in physically restraining aggressive residents. Ten injuries were to the lower extremities, 15 to upper extremities, 8 to the head or neck, and 2 to the back. Four of the injury claims were for bites.

Review of Policies

The center provided no written policies or procedures on workplace violence. Managers reported that direct care staff completed training during new employee orientation and annual training on crisis intervention, which focused on handling agitated behaviors and applying physical restraint. Direct care workers were also required to complete annual training on the following topics: personal safety techniques, behavior management, resident communication skills, and nonviolent crisis management, which included a restraint-reduction effort.

Our review of the ICF/MR regulations showed that the center did not consistently follow these regulations in areas such as

RESULTS

staffing ratios, convening a human rights committee, proper use of medication to manage resident behavior, and staff training.

We reviewed the control plan for bloodborne pathogen exposure because of the bites and other potential exposures to body fluids that direct care workers reported in the interviews and on the OSHA Logs. The plan for controlling exposure to bloodborne pathogens included the basic elements of OSHA's bloodborne pathogen standard, such as for needlestick injuries and handling resident laundry [29 CFR 1910.1030]. Hepatitis B vaccination series were made available for new employees. The plan did not include an evaluation of or prevention strategies related to the infectious disease transmission risk resulting from resident assaults.

DISCUSSION

Incidence rates of overall injury and illness and injury due to assault at the center were higher than national rates in the healthcare and social assistance sector. In addition, the incidence rates of injury and illness increased from 2004 to 2006, with a slight decrease in 2007. Most injuries were from resident assault. The Department of Justice National Crime Victimization Survey Report for 1993–1999 reported rates of simple assault by occupational category, which can offer some comparison [DOJ 2001]. Of the occupational groups in healthcare with the highest average annual rate of simple assault, the survey found that mental health staff experienced 4.3 assaults per 100 workers and nursing staff experienced 2.2 assaults per 100 workers. At 24.7 per 100 workers, the average rate of injury from assault at the center for 2004–2007 was much higher than these rates. However, incidence rates of injuries due to assault were below rates found in a 2004 study at a public ICF/MR in Idaho. In that facility, the average rate of injury among direct healthcare staff was 32.7 per 100 workers [Manning 2005]. We found that most staff did not take days off work after assaults, but of those staff who did, the total amount of lost work time from 2004 through 2008 was more than 3,000 days. Staff who required time off had typically experienced severe injuries that may have required prolonged recovery and treatment.

Every staff member interviewed reported being repeatedly injured by residents and that work-related injuries from resident aggression had been increasing. The types of assaults that staff reported are typical of those documented in other social service and healthcare settings, such as being kicked, hit, bitten, and scratched [NIOSH 2002a]. Most staff reported being injured while physically restraining a resident.

Research has demonstrated that a common adverse consequence of using physical restraint is agitation and that combative residents often become more combative when restrained [Tinetti et al. 1991; Mion and Strumpf 1994; Driscoll 1999; Castle and Engberg 2009].

Workplace violence against staff is common in healthcare and social service settings [Islam et al. 2003; Gerberich et al. 2004; McPhaul 2004; Gerberich et al. 2005; Nachreiner et al. 2007]. Healthcare leads all other industries in the number of nonfatal assaults resulting in lost work days in the United States, accounting for 60% of all such assaults. Nurses, nurse aides, and orderlies had the highest proportion of these injuries [BLS 2007]. However, little is known specifically about the extent of workplace violence against healthcare staff who care for residents with developmental disabilities in long-term care facilities. Most ICF/MRs in the United States, including this center, serve a mix of developmentally disabled, mentally ill, or dually diagnosed residents. Many of these facilities serve residents who have no other placement option because of severe behavioral or medical issues. This situation places direct care workers at higher risk for injury than other healthcare professionals.

A survey that examined the distribution of residents in several U.S. public ICF/MRs showed that 80% of these facilities characterized a portion of their resident population as being dangerous or aggressive and reported that this portion is increasing [Manning 2005]. Working with patients or clients with a known history of assaultive behavior has been identified as a risk factor for hospital employees [NIOSH 2002a]. Persons with mental and physical disabilities may become agitated by certain stressors—including lack of privacy, minimal control over daily activities, and noise level—and have reduced impulse control, which may result in agitation and aggression [Myers et al. 2005; Privitera et al. 2005].

We observed certain aspects of the physical environment and deficiencies in the security system that placed staff at increased risk for injury from assault. Furniture placement was crowded, which could have led to entrapment of staff and inability to observe residents in all areas of the room. Residents could have used some moveable items to assault staff. PPDs were not reliable, so other staff members would not always know to assist in a crisis. Inadequate security and poor environmental controls are associated with increased risk of assault in hospitals and may be significant factors in social services workplaces as well [NIOSH 2002a].

Understaffing may have led to fewer staff being available to assist with resident care and respond in a crisis. In addition, most direct care workers and nurses interviewed reported working overtime (an additional 8-hour shift) during each 1-week period, and 50% reported that overtime was mandatory. Facilities employing healthcare workers are mainly 24-hour, 7-day operations that require working more than 8 hours a day and working night shifts [Lipscomb et al. 2002; Lamberg 2004; NIOSH 2004]. Studies have found that overtime increases fatigue and stress and decreases alertness and job performance, putting employees at greater risk of resident assault and injury [Rogers 1997; Simpson and Severson 2000; Lamberg 2004; Gerberich et al. 2004; Dembe et al. 2005]. Risk of injury has been found to increase every hour after 8 hours of work, and injury risk in the 12th hour of work is twice that in the first 8 hours [Lamberg 2004]. Employees may be less able to react to a resident assault and quickly manage the situation when they are fatigued. Mandatory overtime may limit the worker's ability to plan for sleep and recuperation and to arrange for child care and other family responsibilities. In addition, it has been associated with increased risk of somatic complaints, poor recovery, burnout, and work-home imbalances [Van Der Hulst and Geurts 2001; Golden and Jorgensen 2002; NIOSH 2004]. Direct care staff may be more at risk for injury during the evening, when other staff members—such as psychologists, case managers, and doctors who work traditional business hours—are unavailable to help; however, we did not examine whether work shift was a contributing factor to injury due to assault.

Most staff reported that managers lacked concern about their safety and did not listen to their suggestions about how to handle resident aggression or their input in residents' IPPs. Research has determined that direct care workers have less control over their work environment, fewer opportunities to make independent decisions, and higher levels of job strain than other occupational groups [Karasek and Theorell 1990; Sullivan et al. 1999; Morgan et al. 2002]. In another NIOSH HHE, investigators examined job stress characteristics in employees of a developmental center and found that staff reported one of their most common stressors was having no supervisory support and little control over treatment decisions [NIOSH 2002b]. Organizational factors such as high job strain and low decision latitude have been associated with injuries, cardiovascular disease, and adverse mental health outcomes [Corrigan 1993; Sanne et al. 2005; Schoenfisch and Lipscomb 2009; Rodwell et al. 2009].

DISCUSSION
(CONTINUED)

We found that staff are being assaulted in ways (i.e., bites, scratches, and other injuries that result in broken skin) that could increase risk of bloodborne pathogen transmission, but this was not addressed in the plan for controlling bloodborne pathogen exposure. Hepatitis B virus, human immunodeficiency virus, and hepatitis C virus are the bloodborne pathogens most frequently associated with occupational exposures. In developmental centers, reported staff exposures have been primarily via residents' bites, fingernail scratches, body fluids, and (occasionally) injury from sharp instruments. Staff who are vaccinated are protected from hepatitis B infection, but those assaulted with objects are at risk of tetanus if the assault results in a deep puncture wound or the object is contaminated. The risk that a bloodborne pathogen might be transmitted via fingernail scratches has been reported as minimal, but hepatitis B and hepatitis C can be transmitted via saliva. Transmission of these pathogens to hospital staff with occupational exposure to needlesticks and injuries from other sharps is well documented. A bite poses a risk of infection transmission from the resident to the staff person who is bitten but also vice versa [Lohiya et al. 2001].

This evaluation has several limitations. The injury rates calculated from the OSHA Logs may overestimate or underestimate the extent of this problem. The rates are based on OSHA's basic requirements of recording and reporting only occupational injury and illness events that are severe enough to cause lost work time, require treatment beyond first aid, cause loss of consciousness, or result in restricted work duties or transfer to another job [29 CFR 1904.7]. The rates of less severe injuries and assaults are likely to be much higher; underreporting of injuries and assaults has been reported in other studies [Bensely et al. 1997; Erikson and Williams-Evans 2000; Islam et al. 2003; Myers et al. 2005]. However, some overestimation of rates also may have occurred because the number of overtime hours was not reflected in the formula. To allow comparison with other facilities with the same NAICS code throughout the United States, we used the standard formula number of 200,000 hours, which reflects a standard 40-hour work week. The national incidence rates for nursing and residential facilities and the healthcare and social assistance sector offered the closest comparison with incidence rates of work-related injury and illness and assault at the center, but the industry rate includes employees working in all occupations, some of whom may have lower exposures to the more hazardous aspects of healthcare.

DISCUSSION
(CONTINUED)

In addition, findings from this evaluation apply to this center and may not reflect the injury/assault experiences at other ICF/MRs nationwide. The information from the interviews may not be representative of all direct care staff at this entire facility. The staff members volunteering to participate in our interviews may have been more concerned about resident aggression and as a result may have overestimated the concerns of all direct care staff. We attempted to overcome this issue by serially selecting staff to interview; however, interviews were voluntary, and a few staff declined participation.

CONCLUSIONS

Direct care and nursing staff at this ICF/MR were at risk of injury from assault by residents. Nonfatal injury and illness rates for direct care staff and nurses were much higher than national rates, and injury assault rates were higher than for other healthcare worker groups.

RECOMMENDATIONS

The following recommendations are based on the findings of our site visit to this center. Although the center is now closed, consistent application of these actions should help prevent or reduce resident assault and create a more healthful workplace at any ICF/MR or other similar facility.

Policies

- Develop a proactive safety and health program. This comprehensive program should include management and employee participation; hazard identification; safety and health training; and hazard prevention, control, and reporting.

- To develop a safety and health program, use the State Operations Manual, Interpretive Guidelines—Responsibilities of Intermediate Care Facilities for Persons with Mental Retardation ("Interpretive Guidelines for ICF/MR") and OSHA's Guidelines for Preventing Workplace Violence for Health Care & Social Service Workers ("OSHA Workplace Violence Guidelines"), which are available on the OSHA website at http://www.osha.gov/Publications/OSHA3148/osha3148.html [42 CFR 440.150-480; OSHA 2004].

- Develop a workplace violence prevention policy, using the OSHA Workplace Violence Guidelines. Use this policy to create a culture of safety (including a clear policy of zero tolerance for workplace violence). Once all levels of staff work together to develop this policy, the safety committee should take charge of maintaining safety and promoting the policy.

- Ensure that the bloodborne pathogen policy includes an evaluation of all occupational exposures that could result in infectious disease transmission. This includes all assaults such as bites or puncture wounds in which staff are at risk for disease transmission from infectious body fluids. Explain possible controls to reduce or eliminate such exposures in the exposure control plan, to comply with OSHA's bloodborne pathogen standard [29 CFR 1910.1030].

Physical Environment and Security Measures

- Ensure that staff have access to alarm devices or cell phones where risk is apparent or may be anticipated. Ensure that an adequate number of trained personnel are available to respond to incidents when an alarm is triggered.

Healthcare Management

- Encourage employees to report assaults to their supervisors and seek a prompt referral to a healthcare provider if injury occurs; ensure the provider is experienced in evaluating and treating work-related injuries.

- Require staff to report every incident of assault, even if the event is unlikely to recur or seems minor. Consistently record and follow up cases of injuries from assaults on OSHA Logs and other incident reporting systems as appropriate, to analyze trends and to track the magnitude and seriousness of resident assaults. Incident reporting should include details of the characteristics of attacker and victims, an account of what happened before and during the incident, and the relevant details of the situation and its outcome. Use these findings to look for patterns of incidents and to revise safety procedures when needed.

Safety Committee

- Create a permanent safety committee that uses the OSHA Workplace Violence Guidelines to guide its actions. The committee should consist of all levels and types of staff (especially management, direct care staff, and maintenance employees), who work together to proactively address safety concerns that affect staff and residents. Provide this committee with the resources and management support it needs to implement its recommendations.

Human Rights

- Create a permanent human rights committee in accordance with standard 483.440(f)(3) of the Interpretive Guidelines for ICF/MR [42 CFR 440.15–480].

- Ensure that the committee reviews and approves any resident programs that use restrictive techniques such as restraints/ physical interventions and medications to manage behavior. In addition, ensure that the committee periodically reviews/ monitors such programs to determine whether continued use is justified.

- Re-evaluate the behavior medication policy to ensure that it is being implemented in accordance with the Interpretive Guidelines for ICF/MR [42 CFR 440.15–480].

Staff Scheduling

- Maintain staff–to-resident ratios that meet all applicable requirements (e.g., Interpretive Guidelines for ICF/MR, OSHA requirements, best practices), and exceed these requirements where indicated by residents' IPPs, staff and resident safety requirements, and other relevant concerns.

- Decrease the amount of overtime for direct care workers and nurses, and consider developing a system to reward employees who volunteer for overtime when it is needed.

Training

- Conduct a comprehensive needs assessment to determine training needs.

- Provide regular, ongoing, interactive training as indicated by the needs assessment, Interpretive Guidelines for ICF/MR, and the OSHA Workplace Violence Guidelines for direct care workers and nurses.

Employee Health and Wellness

- Encourage and emphasize employee positive health and wellness programs such as stress management, weight control, smoking cessation, and healthy eating habits.

- Publicize the Employee Service Program; ensure that employees know that this confidential, free program is available to them, and encourage them to use it.

- Develop an effective post-incident response and evaluation program to assist direct care staff and others in dealing with psychological trauma, fear of returning to work, and other consequences of being assaulted and/or injured at work [OSHA 2004].

- Hold monthly group discussions for staff to encourage them to discuss their concerns about residents' day-to-day care and aggressive behavior, as well concerns about their own health and safety.

- Continue to offer crisis intervention services, such as the Traumatic Incident Stress Management Program offered through the state of Michigan for employees who have recently experienced an assault.

- Provide tetanus/diphtheria vaccination to employees in accordance with the Advisory Committee on Immunization Practices.

REFERENCES

Bensley L, Nelson N, Kaufman J, Silverstein B, Kalat J, Shields JW [1997]. Injuries due to assault on psychiatric hospital employees in Washington State. Am J Ind Med 31(1):92–99.

Bureau of Labor Statistics [2007]. Nonfatal occupational injuries and illnesses requiring days away from work, 2006. Washington, DC: U.S. Department of Labor, p. 44.

Castle NG, Engberg J [2009]. The health consequences of using physical restraints in nursing homes. Med Care 47(11):1164–1173.

REFERENCES
(CONTINUED)

CFR. Code of Federal Regulations. Washington, DC: U.S. Government Printing Office, Office of the Federal Register.

Corrigan PW [1993]. Staff stressors at a developmental center and state hospital. Ment Retard 31(4):234–238.

Dembe AE, Erickson JB, Delbos RG, Banks SM [2005]. The impact of overtime and long work hours on occupational injuries and illnesses: new evidence from the United States. Occup Environ Med 62(9):588–597.

Driscoll G [1999]. Restraints in the acute care setting. Advance for Nurses 1(8):11–13.

DOJ [2001]. National Crime Victimization Survey, Violence in the Workplace, 1993–99; U.S. Department of Justice, Office of Justice Programs, Bureau of Justice Statistics Special Report. Washington, DC: U.S. Department of Justice.

Erickson L, Williams-Evans SA [2000]. Attitudes of emergency nurses regarding patient assaults. J Emerg Nurse 26(3):210–215.

Gerberich SG, Church TR, McGovern PM, Hansen H, Nachreiner NM, Geisser MS, Ryan AD, Mongin SJ, Watt GD [2004]. An epidemiological study of the magnitude and consequences of work related violence: the Minnesota Nurses' Study. Occup Environ Med 61(6):495–503.

Gerberich S G, Church TR, McGovern PM, Hansen H, Nachreiner NM, Geisser MS, Ryan AD, Mongin SJ, Watt GD, Jurek A [2005]. Risk factors for work-related assaults on nurses. Epidemiology 16(5):704–709.

Golden L, Jorgensen H [2002]. Time after time: mandatory overtime in the U.S. economy. Economic Policy Institute Briefing Paper #120 [http://www.epi.org/publications/entry/briefingpapers_bp120/]. Date accessed: December 2010.

Islam SS, Edla SR, Mujuru P, Doyle EJ, Ducatman AM [2003]. Risk factors for physical assault: state-managed workers' compensation experience. Am J Prev Med 25(1):31–37.

Karasek J, Theorell T [1990]. Healthy work: stress, productivity and the reconstruction of working life. New York: Basic Books, pp 31–81.

Lamberg L [2004]. Impact of long working hours explored. JAMA 292(1):25–26.

Lipscomb JA, Trinkoff AM, Geiger-Brown J, Brady B [2002]. Work-schedule characteristics and reported musculoskeletal disorders of registered nurses. Scand J Work Environ Health 28(6):394–401.

Lohiya G, Tan-Figueroa L, Lohiya S [2001]. Bloodborne pathogen exposures in a developmental center. Infect Control Hosp Epidemiol 22(6): 8–11.

Manning S [2005]. Injury among direct healthcare staff, an unheralded occupational safety and health crisis. Professional Safety, Journal of the American Society of Safety Engineers [http://www.asse.org/professionalsafety/]. Date accessed: December 2010.

McPhaul KM, Lipscomb JA [2004]. Workplace violence in health care: recognized but not regulated. Online J Issues Nurs 9(3):7.

Mion LC, Strumpf N [1994]. Use of physical restraints in the acute care setting: implications for the nurse. Geriatric Nursing 15(1): 127–132.

Morgan DG, Semchuck KM, Stewart NJ, D'Arcy C [2002]. Job strain among rural nursing homes: a comparison of nurses, aides, and activity workers. J Nurs Adm 32 (3): 152–161.

Myers D, Kriebel D, Kerasek R, Punnett L, Wegman D [2005]. Injuries and assaults in a long-term psychiatric care facility: an epidemiologic study. AAOHN J 53(11):489–498.

Nachreiner NM, Gerberich SG, Ryan AD, McGovern PM [2007]. Minnesota nurses' study: perceptions of violence and the work environment. Ind Health 45(5):672–678.

NIOSH [2002a]. Violence: occupational hazards in hospitals. Cincinnati, OH: U.S. Department of Health and Human Services, Centers for Disease Control and Prevention, National Institute for Occupational Safety and Health, DHHS (NIOSH) Publication No. 2002–101.

NIOSH [2002b]. Health hazard evaluation report: Jergens Road Adult Services Center, Dayton, OH. Cincinnati, OH: U.S. Department of Health and Human Services, Centers for Disease Control and Prevention, National Institute for Occupational Safety and Health, NIOSH HETA No. 2002-0218-2881.

NIOSH [2004]. Overtime and extended work shifts: recent findings in illnesses, injuries and health behaviors. Cincinnati, OH: U.S. Department of Health and Human Services, Centers for Disease

Control and Prevention, National Institute for Occupational Safety and Health, DHHS (NIOSH) Publication No. 2004-143.

OSHA [2004]. Guidelines for preventing workplace violence for health care & social service workers [http://www.osha.gov/Publications/OSHA3148/osha3148.html]. Date accessed: February 2011.

Privitera MR, Weisman R, Cerulli C, Tu X, Groman A [2005]. Violence toward mental health staff and safety in the work environment. Occup Med (Lond) 55(6):480-486.

Rodwell J, Noblet A, Demir D, Steane P [2009]. The impact of the work conditions of allied health professional on satisfaction, commitment, and psychological distress. Health Care Manage Rev 34(3):273-283.

Rogers B [1997]. Health hazards in nursing and health care: an overview. Am J Infect Control 25(3):248-261.

Sanne B, Mykletun A, Dahl AA, Moen BE, Tell GS [2005]. Testing the job demand-control support model with anxiety and depression as outcomes: the Hordaland Health Study. Occup Med (Lond) 55(6):463-473.

Schoenfisch AL, Lipscomb HJ [2009]. Job characteristics and work organization factors associated with patient-handling injury among nursing personnel. Work 33(1):117-128.

Simpson CL, Severson RK [2000]. Risk of injury in African American hospital workers. J Occup Environ Med 42(10):1035-1040.

Sullivan T, Kerr M, Ibrahim S [1999]. Job stress in healthcare workers: highlights from the National Population Health Survey. Hosp Q 2(4):34-40.

Tinetti ME, Liu W, Marottoli RA, Ginter SF [1991]. Mechanical restraint use among residents of skilled nursing facilities. JAMA 265(4):468-471.

Van Der Hulst M, Geurts S [2001]. Associations between overtime and psychological health in high and low reward jobs. Work Stress 15:227-240.

ACKNOWLEDGMENTS AND AVAILABILITY OF REPORT

The Hazard Evaluations and Technical Assistance Branch (HETAB) of the National Institute for Occupational Safety and Health (NIOSH) conducts field investigations of possible health hazards in the workplace. These investigations are conducted under the authority of Section 20(a)(6) of the Occupational Safety and Health (OSHA) Act of 1970, 29 U.S.C. 669(a)(6), which authorizes the Secretary of Health and Human Services, following a written request from any employer or authorized representative of employees, to determine whether any substance normally found in the place of employment has potentially toxic effects in such concentrations as used or found. HETAB also provides, upon request, technical and consultative assistance to federal, state, and local agencies; labor; industry; and other groups or individuals to control occupational health hazards and to prevent related trauma and disease.

The findings and conclusions in this report are those of the authors and do not necessarily represent the views of NIOSH. Mention of any company or product does not constitute endorsement by NIOSH. In addition, citations to websites external to NIOSH do not constitute NIOSH endorsement of the sponsoring organizations or their programs or products. Furthermore, NIOSH is not responsible for the content of these websites. All Web addresses referenced in this document were accessible as of the publication date.

This report was prepared by Christine West and Ellen Galloway of HETAB, Division of Surveillance, Hazard Evaluations and Field Studies. Field assistance was provided by Gricelda Gomez. Health communication assistance was provided by Stefanie Evans. Editorial assistance was provided by Seleen Collins. Desktop publishing was performed by Robin Smith.

Copies of this report have been sent to employee and management representatives at Michigan Department of Community Health and the OSHA Regional Office. This report is not copyrighted and may be freely reproduced. The report may be viewed and printed at www.cdc.gov/niosh/hhe/. Copies may be purchased from the National Technical Information Service, at 5825 Port Royal Road, Springfield, Virginia 22161.

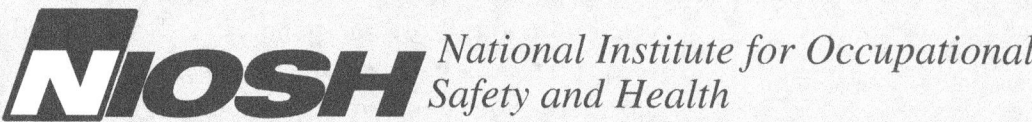
National Institute for Occupational Safety and Health

Delivering on the Nation's promise: Safety and health at work for all people through research and prevention.

To receive NIOSH documents or information about occupational safety and health topics, contact NIOSH at:

1-800-CDC-INFO (1-800-232-4636)

TTY: 1-888-232-6348

E-mail: cdcinfo@cdc.gov

or visit the NIOSH web site at: **www.cdc.gov/niosh.**

For a monthly update on news at NIOSH, subscribe to NIOSH eNews by visiting **www.cdc.gov/niosh/eNews.**

SAFER • HEALTHIER • PEOPLE™